Table Of Contents

Chapter 1: Understanding Addiction

The Impact of Addiction on Mothers

Motherhood is a beautiful journey filled with love, joy, and nurturing. However, for mothers battling addiction, this journey can quickly turn into a nightmare. The impact of addiction on mothers is profound and far-reaching, affecting not only their own lives but also the lives of their children and families. In this subchapter, we will explore the various aspects of this impact and provide guidance and support for moms in recovery.

For children, having a mother who is addicted to drugs or alcohol can be incredibly challenging. They may witness erratic behavior, neglect, and even abuse. The emotional toll on these children can be immense, leading to anxiety, depression, and a range of other psychological issues. In this section, we will delve into coping strategies for children with addicted parents, offering practical tips and resources to help them navigate this difficult terrain.

Recovery is a journey, and for mothers in recovery, it takes on a unique set of challenges. In this subchapter, we will discuss addiction recovery programs specifically tailored for mothers. These programs recognize the importance of addressing the specific needs and responsibilities of mothers, such as childcare and household management. We will provide a comprehensive list of resources and programs that cater to these needs, ensuring that mothers have the support they require to successfully overcome addiction.

Legal and custody issues can be particularly complex for mothers in recovery. Co-parenting with an addicted mother presents a host of challenges, including concerns about the safety and well-being of the child. In this section, we will delve into the legal and custody issues surrounding co-parenting with an addicted mother, providing guidance on navigating these difficult waters. We will address topics such as establishing a custody agreement, ensuring the child's safety, and seeking legal recourse when necessary.

This subchapter is an essential resource for moms in recovery, offering guidance, support, and practical strategies for navigating the impact of addiction on mothers. It is a beacon of hope, reminding mothers that recovery is possible and that they have the strength and resilience to rebuild their lives and heal their families. By addressing the unique challenges faced by moms in recovery, we hope to empower them to overcome addiction and create a brighter future for themselves and their children.

The Cycle of Addiction and Recovery

In the journey of addiction and recovery, understanding the cycle of addiction is crucial for moms who are on the path to recovery. This subchapter explores the intricate cycle of addiction and the steps involved in the recovery process, offering guidance and support to moms in recovery.

The cycle of addiction is a pattern that individuals struggling with addiction often experience. It starts with the initial experimentation or use, which may seem harmless and recreational. However, for some, this casual use can quickly spiral into regular or even daily use. As addiction takes hold, the individual begins to experience negative consequences, such as strained relationships, health issues, or legal problems.

For moms in recovery, understanding the cycle of addiction can help them recognize the signs and symptoms of their own addiction. By identifying the stages of the cycle, they can interrupt the pattern and take proactive steps towards their recovery journey. It is important for moms to realize that addiction is not a moral failing, but rather a complex disease that requires professional help and support.

In this subchapter, we delve into coping strategies for children with addicted parents. We understand that addiction not only affects the individual but also has a profound impact on their loved ones, especially children. We provide insights and practical techniques to help moms in recovery navigate the challenges of parenting while healing from addiction.

Additionally, we explore addiction recovery programs specifically tailored for mothers. These programs address the unique needs and circumstances faced by moms in recovery, including child care, parenting skills, and rebuilding trust with their children. We highlight the importance of seeking professional help and participating in support groups to ensure a successful recovery journey.

Furthermore, legal and custody issues in co-parenting with an addicted mother are discussed in detail. We provide valuable information on navigating the legal system, ensuring the well-being of children, and establishing healthy co-parenting relationships. Our aim is to empower moms in recovery to overcome legal challenges and create a safe and supportive environment for their children.

"The Cycle of Addiction and Recovery" subchapter is a comprehensive guide for moms in recovery, addressing their unique challenges and providing the necessary tools to break free from addiction. It offers hope, support, and practical strategies for moms to rebuild their lives and create a better future for themselves and their children.

Common Signs and Symptoms of Addiction

Recognizing the signs and symptoms of addiction is crucial for moms in recovery, as it enables them to identify if they or their loved ones are struggling with addiction. By understanding these indicators, moms can take the necessary steps to seek help and support. In this subchapter, we will explore the common signs and symptoms of addiction, providing valuable insights for moms in recovery.

1. Physical and Behavioral Changes: Addiction often leads to noticeable physical and behavioral changes. Moms may experience weight loss or gain, changes in sleep patterns, and neglect of personal hygiene. They may also exhibit mood swings, become secretive, isolate themselves from loved ones, or experience financial difficulties due to their addictive behaviors.

2. Strong Cravings and Loss of Control: One of the key signs of addiction is an intense craving for the substance or behavior. Moms may find themselves preoccupied with obtaining and using the addictive substance, often resulting in a loss of control over their actions and priorities.

3. Tolerance and Withdrawal: Over time, individuals with addiction develop a tolerance, requiring higher doses or more frequent engagement in the addictive behavior to achieve the same effect. When they stop using the substance or engaging in the behavior, withdrawal symptoms may occur, such as anxiety, irritability, insomnia, or physical discomfort.

4. Neglect of Responsibilities: Addiction can cause moms to neglect their responsibilities, both at home and work. They may struggle to fulfill their role as a parent, leading to a decline in childcare, household management, and overall family functioning.

5. Relationship Issues: Addiction often strains relationships, causing conflicts and breakdowns in communication. Moms may experience difficulties in maintaining healthy relationships with their children, partners, or co-parents. Children may suffer emotionally and struggle with trust, stability, and attachment issues.

Recognizing these signs and symptoms of addiction is the first step towards seeking help and recovery. As moms in recovery, it is essential to remember that addiction is a treatable disease, and there are tailored addiction recovery programs available specifically designed to support mothers. Additionally, legal and custody issues in co-parenting with an addicted mother can be addressed through legal assistance and support networks.

By understanding these common signs and symptoms, moms in recovery can take proactive steps towards their own healing and create a healthier environment for their children. Remember, seeking help is a sign of strength, and with the right support, recovery is possible.

Chapter 2: My Daughter's Mom is a Junkie

Recognizing the Impact on Children

As moms in recovery, it is crucial for us to acknowledge the profound impact our addiction has had on our children. Our journey towards recovery not only involves healing ourselves but also creating a safe and nurturing environment for our children to thrive in. In this subchapter, we will explore the various ways addiction affects our children and provide guidance on how to support them through their own healing process.

"My daughter's mom is a junkie" is a painful reality that many children face when their mothers struggle with addiction. The stigma attached to addiction can make it challenging for children to understand and cope with their mother's behavior. We will discuss how best to address this issue with empathy and honesty, helping our children comprehend the reasons behind our addiction and reassuring them that it is not their fault.

Coping strategies for children with addicted parents are essential tools for both us and our children. We will explore effective ways to support our children emotionally, providing them with a safe space to express their feelings. By understanding their unique needs, we can help them develop healthy coping mechanisms and empower them to navigate the challenges they may face as a result of our addiction.

Addiction recovery programs specifically tailored for mothers offer a lifeline for us on our journey towards recovery. These programs provide not only the necessary tools for overcoming addiction but also address the specific needs and challenges we face as mothers. We will explore the various resources available, from inpatient treatment centers to outpatient support groups, that can help us regain control of our lives while still fulfilling our roles as mothers. Legal and custody issues in co-parenting with an addicted mother can be complex and overwhelming. We will delve into the legal aspects of co-parenting and provide guidance on how to navigate custody arrangements, visitation rights, and court proceedings. By understanding our legal rights and responsibilities, we can work towards establishing a healthy co-parenting relationship that prioritizes the well-being of our children.

Recognizing the impact our addiction has had on our children is the first step towards healing. By addressing their emotional needs, seeking tailored recovery programs, and navigating legal and custody issues, we can create a stable and loving environment that supports their growth and well-being. Together, we can overcome the challenges of addiction and rebuild the bonds with our children, fostering a brighter future for both ourselves and our loved ones.

Communicating with Children about Addiction

One of the most challenging aspects of addiction recovery for mothers is explaining the situation to their children. Addressing the topic of addiction with children requires sensitivity, honesty, and an understanding of their age and emotional development. In this subchapter, we will explore effective ways for moms in recovery to communicate with their children about addiction and provide support to help them cope with the challenges they may face.

When discussing addiction with children, it is important to use age-appropriate language and concepts. Younger children may struggle to understand the complexities of addiction, so it is crucial to keep explanations simple and concrete. For example, you can explain addiction as a sickness that affects the brain and body, making it difficult for someone to make healthy choices. Emphasize that addiction is not a personal failing or a result of their behavior.

Older children may have a better understanding of addiction, but they may also carry feelings of guilt, shame, or confusion. Encourage open and honest conversations, allowing them to express their emotions and ask questions. Assure them that their feelings are valid and provide reassurance that your recovery is not their responsibility.

In addition to open communication, it is essential to implement coping strategies for children with addicted parents. Encourage them to express their emotions through art, writing, or talking to a trusted adult. Provide a safe and stable environment where they can find comfort and support. Consider involving them in support groups or therapy sessions specifically designed for children of addicted parents.

As a mom in recovery, it is crucial to seek addiction recovery programs that are tailored for mothers. These programs can provide a supportive community of other moms facing similar challenges, as well as specialized resources to address the unique needs of mothers in recovery. By participating in these programs, you can gain valuable insights and strategies for maintaining sobriety while effectively parenting your children.

Lastly, legal and custody issues often arise when co-parenting with an addicted mother. It is important to educate yourself about your rights and responsibilities, as well as the potential impact of addiction on custody arrangements. Seek legal advice to ensure that you are taking the necessary steps to protect both yourself and your children.

In conclusion, communicating with children about addiction is a delicate and challenging task for moms in recovery. By utilizing age-appropriate language, providing support, and involving them in specialized programs, you can help your children understand addiction while fostering their emotional well-being. Additionally, addressing legal and custody issues will ensure a safe and stable environment for your children. Remember, you are not alone in this battle, and there are resources available to support you and your family through this journey of recovery.

Helping Children Cope with a Parent's Addiction

Introduction:

As a mother in recovery, one of the most challenging aspects of your journey may be helping your children cope with your addiction. This subchapter aims to provide guidance and strategies to support you in navigating this sensitive issue. By understanding the impact of addiction on children, exploring coping strategies, discovering addiction recovery programs tailored for mothers, and addressing legal and custody issues, you can create a healthier environment for your child's growth and emotional well-being.

Understanding the Impact:

Children of addicted parents often experience a wide range of emotions, including confusion, fear, anger, and sadness. It is crucial to acknowledge their feelings and validate their experiences. By doing so, you can create an environment that encourages open communication and emotional healing.

Coping Strategies for Children with Addicted Parents:

To help your child cope with your addiction, it is essential to establish routines, consistency, and stability in their lives. Providing a safe and nurturing space, engaging in age-appropriate conversations about addiction, and offering them an outlet for expressing their emotions can contribute to their healing process. Additionally, involving them in support groups or counseling can be immensely beneficial.

Addiction Recovery Programs Specifically Tailored for Mothers:

Recognizing the unique challenges faced by mothers in recovery, several addiction recovery programs offer specialized support and resources. These programs cater to the specific needs of mothers, including childcare services, tailored counseling, and educational workshops. Engaging with these programs can provide you with the necessary tools to rebuild your life while prioritizing your responsibilities as a mother.

Legal and Custody Issues in Co-Parenting with an Addicted Mother:

Co-parenting with an addicted mother can present complex legal and custody challenges. It is essential to familiarize yourself with the legal framework surrounding addiction and parenting rights. Seeking legal advice from professionals who specialize in family law and addiction-related issues can help you navigate these complexities and ensure the best interests of your child are protected.

Conclusion:

Helping your children cope with your addiction is a critical part of your recovery journey as a mother. By understanding the impact of addiction on children, implementing coping strategies, engaging in specialized addiction recovery programs for mothers, and addressing legal and custody issues, you can create a nurturing and supportive environment for your child's emotional well-being. Remember, by taking care of yourself and your recovery, you are also taking care of your children, setting the stage for a brighter and healthier future.

Chapter 3: Coping Strategies for Children with Addicted Parents

Creating a Safe and Stable Environment

As mothers in recovery, our primary goal is to provide a safe and stable environment for our children. We understand the challenges that come with addiction and the impact it can have on our little ones. This subchapter aims to guide you on how to create a nurturing space for your children while navigating the ups and downs of recovery.

One of the first steps in creating a safe environment is to establish a routine. Children thrive on predictability, especially when coming from a chaotic past. By setting consistent meal times, bedtimes, and daily activities, you provide a sense of stability that helps them feel secure. Additionally, having a schedule allows you to plan your own recovery activities, therapy sessions, and support group meetings without disrupting their routine.

Open communication is essential in any relationship, but it becomes even more crucial when dealing with addiction. Be honest with your children about your past struggles, in an age-appropriate manner. Let them know that you are in recovery and working towards a healthier life. Encourage them to ask questions and express their feelings, assuring them that their emotions are valid and safe to share.

It's important to acknowledge that children with addicted parents often face unique challenges. They may have experienced trauma or witnessed disturbing events. Coping strategies tailored specifically for these children can help them process their emotions and develop resilience. Explore therapy options or support groups designed for children from addicted families. These resources can provide a safe space for them to express themselves and learn healthy coping mechanisms.

As mothers in recovery, it is vital to take advantage of addiction recovery programs specifically tailored for mothers. These programs understand the unique needs and responsibilities of motherhood and provide a supportive community of fellow moms in recovery. By participating in these programs, you can gain invaluable tools, guidance, and support while creating a strong network of women who understand your journey.

Finally, legal and custody issues may arise when co-parenting with an addicted mother. Educate yourself on the relevant laws and regulations and seek professional advice to ensure the best outcome for your child. It's essential to prioritize their safety and well-being, even if it means making difficult decisions.

Remember, creating a safe and stable environment for your children is a continuous process. It requires dedication, self-reflection, and ongoing growth. By implementing these strategies and seeking support, you are taking crucial steps towards providing your children with the loving and stable environment they deserve.

Building a Support System for Children

As mothers in recovery, one of the most important aspects we need to focus on is building a strong support system for our children. Our journey to overcome addiction is not just about our own recovery; it also involves ensuring the well-being of our children and providing them with the support they need to navigate the challenges that come with having an addicted parent.

When it comes to supporting our children, communication is key. It is crucial to have open and honest conversations with our children about addiction, in an age-appropriate manner. This helps them understand the situation and reduces the stigma associated with addiction. By creating a safe space for our children to express their feelings, we can help them cope with the emotional roller coaster they may be experiencing.

Coping strategies for children with addicted parents are essential to help them navigate the complexities of their lives. Encouraging them to express their emotions through creative outlets such as art, music, or journaling can be incredibly therapeutic. Additionally, connecting them with support groups or counseling services specifically designed for children of addicted parents can provide them with a sense of community and the opportunity to share their experiences with others who can relate.

There are addiction recovery programs specifically tailored for mothers that can play a crucial role in building a support system. These programs not only address our own recovery but also provide resources and guidance on how to support our children throughout the process. They offer a safe environment for us to learn and grow while prioritizing the needs of our children.

Legal and custody issues in co-parenting with an addicted mother can be overwhelming. It is essential to seek legal advice and understand our rights and responsibilities as parents. Maintaining open lines of communication with the other parent, when possible, can help ensure the well-being of our children. Co-parenting with an addicted mother requires setting boundaries, seeking professional help, and prioritizing the best interests of our children.

In conclusion, building a support system for our children is a crucial aspect of our recovery journey as mothers. By fostering open communication, teaching coping strategies, accessing tailored addiction recovery programs, and addressing legal and custody issues, we can provide our children with the support they need to thrive despite the challenges they may face. Remember, we are not alone in this battle, and by prioritizing our children's well-being, we are giving them the best chance at a healthy and fulfilling life.

Teaching Children Healthy Coping Mechanisms

As moms in recovery, one of the most important tasks we have is to help our children navigate the challenging terrain of having an addicted parent. Our children are resilient, but they need our guidance and support to develop healthy coping mechanisms. In this subchapter, we will explore effective strategies to teach our children how to cope with the challenges they may face in their lives.

Children with addicted parents often experience a range of emotions such as fear, anger, confusion, and sadness. It is crucial to create a safe and open space for our children to express these emotions without judgment. Encourage them to talk about their feelings and actively listen to their concerns. Validating their emotions and providing reassurance can help them feel understood and supported.

Another important aspect of teaching healthy coping mechanisms is to model positive behaviors ourselves. Children learn by observing and imitating their parents. When they see us using healthy coping strategies, such as exercising, practicing mindfulness, or engaging in creative activities, they are more likely to adopt these behaviors themselves.

Teaching our children effective problem-solving skills is also essential. Help them identify the challenges they are facing and guide them through the process of finding solutions. Encourage them to brainstorm ideas, weigh the pros and cons of each option, and make informed decisions. By empowering them to take control of their circumstances, we equip them with valuable skills that can serve them well throughout their lives.

Another important aspect to consider is the availability of addiction recovery programs specifically tailored for mothers. These programs not only provide support for our own recovery journey but also offer resources and guidance for parenting in sobriety. By participating in these programs, we can learn new techniques and strategies to help our children cope with the challenges they may face.

Navigating legal and custody issues can be particularly challenging when co-parenting with an addicted mother. It is crucial to seek legal advice and understand our rights and options. By being well-informed, we can better protect our children's well-being and ensure they have a stable and nurturing environment.

In conclusion, as moms in recovery, we have a unique responsibility to teach our children healthy coping mechanisms. By creating a safe and open space for them to express their emotions, modeling positive behaviors, teaching problem-solving skills, and accessing appropriate support systems, we can help our children thrive despite the challenges they may face. Together, we can create a brighter future for ourselves and our children.

Chapter 4: Addiction Recovery Programs Specifically Tailored for Mothers

The Importance of Seeking Help

In the journey of addiction recovery, seeking help is not just an option, but a crucial step towards reclaiming your life and rebuilding your family. As a mom in recovery, you may have experienced the overwhelming weight of addiction and its impact on your relationship with your children. This subchapter aims to emphasize the significance of seeking help and guide you towards resources tailored to your unique circumstances.

For moms in recovery, seeking help is essential for breaking the cycle of addiction and creating a healthier future for yourself and your children. It takes strength and courage to admit that you need assistance, but the rewards are invaluable. By reaching out, you can access the support and guidance necessary to navigate the challenges of addiction recovery while maintaining your role as a loving and responsible mother.

One of the niches addressed in this subchapter is "My daughter's mom is a junkie." If you find yourself in this situation, it is crucial to acknowledge the impact your addiction has on your child. Seeking help demonstrates your commitment to their well-being and offers them a chance to heal from the pain caused by your addiction. By actively engaging in recovery programs, therapy, and support groups, you can rebuild trust and repair the parent-child relationship. Another niche discussed here is "Coping strategies for children with addicted parents." Seeking help not only benefits you but also provides your children with the tools to cope with the challenges they face. Professional guidance can help them understand addiction, express their emotions, and develop healthy coping mechanisms. By seeking help, you are empowering your children to navigate the complexities of having an addicted parent.

This subchapter also explores "Addiction recovery programs specifically tailored for mothers." Recognizing the unique needs of mothers in recovery, specialized programs offer comprehensive support, addressing issues like parenting skills, trauma, and self-care. These programs provide a safe space for mothers to connect, share experiences, and learn from one another, fostering a sense of community and understanding.

Lastly, "Legal and custody issues in co-parenting with an addicted mother" is a niche addressed here. Seeking legal assistance can help you navigate the complexities of co-parenting while in recovery. A lawyer experienced in addiction-related custody issues can guide you through the legal system, ensuring your rights as a mother in recovery are protected and helping you establish a healthy co-parenting relationship.

In conclusion, seeking help is not a sign of weakness but a courageous step towards healing and rebuilding your life as a mom in recovery. By acknowledging the importance of seeking help, you open doors to a brighter future for both yourself and your children. Remember, you are not alone, and there are resources specifically tailored to support you on this journey.

Inpatient vs. Outpatient Programs

As a mom in recovery, it's crucial to understand the different types of addiction recovery programs available to you. Two common options are inpatient and outpatient programs. Both have their own benefits and considerations, so it's important to choose the one that aligns best with your specific needs and circumstances.

Inpatient programs, also known as residential treatment, involve staying at a treatment facility for a designated period. This option provides a structured and immersive environment that minimizes external distractions and triggers. Inpatient programs often offer a range of therapies, including individual counseling, group therapy, and holistic approaches such as yoga and meditation. These programs are intensive and provide around-the-clock support from trained professionals.

For moms facing severe addiction or those who require a higher level of care, inpatient programs can be highly beneficial. They offer a safe and supportive space where you can focus solely on your recovery. Being away from your usual environment can also help break the cycle of addiction and provide a fresh start.

On the other hand, outpatient programs allow you to live at home while attending treatment sessions regularly. These programs offer flexibility, allowing you to continue fulfilling your responsibilities as a mother, such as taking care of your children or maintaining a job. Outpatient programs typically involve counseling sessions, group therapy, and various educational workshops.

While outpatient programs provide more freedom and the ability to maintain your daily routine, they require a higher level of self-discipline and commitment. It's crucial to have a strong support system in place to help you stay on track, especially during challenging moments.

As a mom in recovery, it's essential to consider your unique circumstances, such as your addiction severity, childcare responsibilities, and overall support network, when choosing between inpatient and outpatient programs. Consulting with addiction specialists or counselors can provide valuable guidance in making this decision.

Remember, there is no one-size-fits-all approach to recovery. What matters most is finding a program that suits your individual needs and helps you on your journey towards a healthier, happier life for both you and your children. You deserve support, understanding, and the opportunity to heal.

Therapy and Counseling for Mothers in Recovery

As a mother in recovery, it is crucial to prioritize your mental and emotional well-being. Therapy and counseling can play a vital role in your journey towards healing and rebuilding a healthy life for yourself and your family. In this subchapter, we will explore the importance of therapy and counseling for mothers in recovery and how it can positively impact various aspects of your life.

Recovery from addiction is a complex process that involves not only breaking free from substance abuse but also addressing the underlying issues that contribute to addiction. Therapy provides a safe and confidential space for you to delve into these underlying issues, understand the root causes of your addiction, and develop coping strategies to prevent relapse. A skilled therapist can guide you through this healing process, helping you to regain control over your life and build a solid foundation for a healthier future.

One niche that may find this subchapter particularly relevant is the audience of "My daughter's mom is a junkie." It is crucial for family members and loved ones to understand the importance of therapy for mothers in recovery. By seeking therapy, mothers can rebuild trust, repair relationships, and create a nurturing environment for their children. Therapy can also help children cope with the challenges of having addicted parents, as discussed in the niche of "Coping strategies for children with addicted parents." By addressing their emotions and providing them with the necessary support, therapy can significantly improve the well-being of both mothers and their children.

Additionally, this subchapter will explore addiction recovery programs specifically tailored for mothers. These programs understand the unique challenges that mothers face in their recovery journey, such as balancing childcare responsibilities, addressing legal and custody issues, and navigating co-parenting with an addicted mother. By participating in these specialized programs, mothers can receive the support they need to overcome these challenges and build a healthier and more stable life for themselves and their children.

Lastly, legal and custody issues are a significant concern for mothers in recovery. This subchapter will touch upon the potential legal and custody issues that may arise when co-parenting with an addicted mother. It will provide guidance on navigating these challenges and seeking legal assistance when necessary to protect the best interests of both the mother and the child.

In conclusion, therapy and counseling are crucial components of a mother's recovery journey. They provide a safe space for healing, help rebuild relationships, and equip mothers with the tools needed to navigate the unique challenges they face. By seeking therapy, mothers can improve their own well-being while also creating a positive and nurturing environment for their children.

Chapter 5: Legal and Custody Issues in Co-Parenting with an Addicted Mother

Understanding Legal Rights and Responsibilities

When it comes to addiction recovery, it is essential for moms to be aware of their legal rights and responsibilities. Navigating the legal system can be overwhelming, but having a clear understanding of your rights and responsibilities can empower you to make informed decisions that are in the best interest of both you and your child. This subchapter aims to provide valuable insights and guidance for moms in recovery as they face legal and custody issues while co-parenting with an addicted mother.

One of the primary concerns for moms in recovery is how addiction affects their custody and visitation rights. It's crucial to be aware that addiction can impact custody decisions, but it doesn't automatically mean that you will lose custody of your child. The court's primary focus is always the child's best interest, and if you can demonstrate your commitment to recovery and provide a stable and safe environment for your child, you have a strong chance of retaining custody or obtaining visitation rights.

To protect your legal rights and strengthen your case, it is essential to document your recovery journey. Keep records of your participation in addiction recovery programs specifically tailored for mothers, therapy sessions, and any other activities that demonstrate your commitment to sobriety and being a responsible parent. This documentation can serve as valuable evidence in court and help you present a compelling argument for custody or visitation rights.

Co-parenting with an addicted mother can be challenging, but understanding your legal rights and responsibilities can help you navigate this complex situation. It is crucial to establish clear boundaries and communication channels with the other parent to ensure the safety and well-being of your child. Seek legal advice to understand your rights in terms of decision-making, visitation schedules, and potential modifications to custody arrangements.

Additionally, it is essential to be aware of the coping strategies for children with addicted parents. Your child may experience a range of emotions and challenges due to their parent's addiction. By proactively seeking resources and support, such as counseling or support groups for children of addicted parents, you can help your child navigate their feelings and develop healthy coping mechanisms.

Remember, you are not alone in this battle. Reach out to support networks, such as community organizations or addiction recovery programs, that specifically cater to mothers in recovery. These programs can provide you with invaluable guidance, legal resources, and emotional support throughout your journey.

Understanding your legal rights and responsibilities as a mom in recovery is crucial for navigating the complexities of co-parenting with an addicted mother. By being informed, proactive, and seeking the necessary support, you can create a safe and stable environment for yourself and your child, ensuring their well-being and your continued recovery.

Navigating the Custody Process

When it comes to co-parenting with an addicted mother, the custody process can be a challenging and complex journey. As a mom in recovery, it is crucial to be well-informed and prepared to ensure the best outcome for yourself and your children. This subchapter aims to provide you with valuable insights and guidance to help you navigate the custody process successfully.

Legal and custody issues in co-parenting with an addicted mother can be overwhelming, but understanding the process is the first step. It is essential to consult with an experienced family law attorney who specializes in addiction-related cases. They can guide you through the legalities, explain your rights, and help you develop a strong case.

In co-parenting situations where the other parent is struggling with addiction, it's imperative to focus on the well-being of your children. Coping strategies for children with addicted parents are vital for their emotional and mental stability. Encourage open communication, create a safe environment, and consider seeking professional counseling or support groups. Helping your children understand addiction without demonizing their other parent is crucial for their healing process.

Addiction recovery programs specifically tailored for mothers can provide you with the tools, support, and resources needed to navigate the custody process effectively. Seek out programs that address the unique challenges faced by moms in recovery, such as childcare assistance, parenting skills development, and relapse prevention strategies. These programs can not only strengthen your case but also enhance your personal growth as a mother in recovery.

Co-parenting with an addicted mother requires a delicate balance between advocating for your children's safety and the rights of the other parent. The court may order drug testing, supervised visitation, or even custody modifications based on the evidence presented. Keep detailed records of any concerning behavior, missed visitations, or instances where your children's safety is compromised. This documentation can be crucial during the custody process.

Remember, the ultimate goal is to create a healthy and stable environment for your children. Be proactive, stay informed, and prioritize their well-being. By focusing on your own recovery, seeking professional support, and understanding the legalities involved, you can navigate the custody process with confidence and strength.

In conclusion, the custody process can be daunting for moms in recovery who are co-parenting with an addicted mother. However, by utilizing coping strategies for children, seeking addiction recovery programs tailored for mothers, understanding the legalities, and advocating for your children's safety, you can ensure the best outcome for all involved. Remember, you are not alone in this battle, and there is support available to help you navigate through these challenging times.

Co-Parenting Strategies for Mothers in Recovery

Introduction:
Co-parenting can be challenging under normal circumstances, but when a mother is in recovery from addiction, it can present a unique set of difficulties. This subchapter aims to provide strategies and guidance for mothers in recovery who are navigating the complexities of co-parenting. Whether you are concerned about your child's well-being, seeking support for your own recovery, or dealing

with legal and custody issues, this chapter will provide valuable insights and coping strategies.

1. Prioritize Open Communication:

Effective co-parenting requires open and honest communication. Establishing regular and respectful communication channels with your child's other parent is vital. Keep the lines of communication open, sharing relevant information about your recovery journey and progress. This will help build trust and foster a healthier co-parenting relationship.

2. Seek Support:

Recovery can be an ongoing process, and having a strong support system is crucial. Connect with addiction recovery programs specifically tailored for mothers. These programs provide a safe space to share experiences, gain insights, and receive guidance from professionals who understand the unique challenges faced by mothers in recovery. Surround yourself with positive influences that will support your journey towards sobriety and successful co-parenting.

3. Address the Needs of Your Child:

Recognize that your child may have unique emotional needs due to your addiction and subsequent recovery. Seek resources and coping strategies for children with addicted parents. Encourage open dialogue with your child, ensuring they feel safe and comfortable sharing their feelings. Consider family therapy sessions as a way to address any underlying issues and help your child cope with the challenges they may face.

4. Legal and Custody Issues:

Navigating legal and custody issues can be overwhelming. Consult with professionals who specialize in family law, particularly those experienced in dealing with addiction-related cases. Educate yourself on your rights as a mother in recovery, and seek legal advice to ensure you are making informed decisions that prioritize the well-being of both you and your child.

Conclusion:

Co-parenting as a mother in recovery poses unique challenges, but with the right strategies and support, it is possible to establish a healthy and successful co-parenting relationship. Prioritizing open communication, seeking support from tailored recovery programs, addressing your child's needs, and navigating legal and custody issues will help you navigate this challenging journey. Remember, your recovery is a gift to both yourself and your child, and by focusing on your well-being, you are also providing a positive example for them.

Chapter 6: Rebuilding Relationships in Recovery

Healing and Reconnecting with Children

As a mom in recovery, one of the most important steps on your journey is healing and reconnecting with your children. Addiction can take a toll on the parent-child relationship, but with the right strategies and support, you can rebuild trust and create a healthy and loving bond with your children once again.

For moms whose children have witnessed their addiction firsthand, it's essential to acknowledge the impact it has had on them. Many children of addicted parents experience a range of emotions, including fear, anger, confusion, and sadness. They may blame themselves or feel abandoned, and it's crucial to address these feelings in a safe and nurturing way.

Coping strategies for children with addicted parents can help them navigate their emotions and begin the healing process. Open and honest communication is key, allowing children to express their feelings and ask questions without judgment. Age-appropriate explanations about addiction can help them understand that it is not their fault and that you are taking steps to recover.

In addition to communication, addiction recovery programs specifically tailored for mothers can provide invaluable support. These programs often offer parenting classes and counseling services, helping moms develop the skills needed to rebuild their relationships with their children. By working on your own recovery, you are also setting a positive example for your children and showing them the importance of perseverance and self-care.

Legal and custody issues in co-parenting with an addicted mother can be challenging, but it's vital to prioritize the well-being of your children. Seeking legal advice and mediation services can help you navigate the complexities of co-parenting while in recovery. By establishing clear boundaries and adhering to court orders, you can create stability and consistency for your children.

Remember, healing and reconnecting with your children is a process that takes time and patience. It's essential to be gentle with yourself and understand that rebuilding trust may not happen overnight. However, with dedication, love, and support, you can create a new and healthy chapter in your relationship with your children.

"The Addiction Battle: A Guide for Moms in Recovery" provides additional guidance and resources to assist you on this journey. By addressing the specific challenges faced by moms in recovery, this book offers practical advice and encouragement to help you heal, reconnect, and create a brighter future for both you and your children.

Rebuilding Trust with Loved Ones

One of the most challenging aspects of addiction recovery is rebuilding trust with loved ones. For moms in recovery, this process is especially crucial as the well-being of their children and co-parenting relationships are at stake. In this subchapter, we will explore effective strategies to rebuild trust and mend relationships with loved ones.

For moms whose children have witnessed their struggle with addiction, it is essential to address their concerns and fears head-on. Children may feel confused, angry, or even blame themselves for their mother's addiction. Open and honest communication is key in helping children understand that addiction is a disease and not their fault. Providing age-appropriate explanations and reassurances can help alleviate their anxieties and create a foundation for rebuilding trust.

Coping strategies for children with addicted parents are also crucial in this process. As a mom in recovery, it is important to be proactive in seeking resources and support for your children. This could include therapy, support groups, or educational materials specifically tailored for children of addicted parents. By addressing their emotional needs and teaching them healthy coping mechanisms, you can help them navigate the challenges they may face.

Addiction recovery programs specifically tailored for mothers can be a valuable resource in rebuilding trust. These programs understand the unique challenges faced by moms in recovery and provide a supportive environment where they can heal and learn new skills. By actively participating in these programs, moms can demonstrate their commitment to sobriety and gain valuable tools to rebuild trust with their loved ones.

Legal and custody issues in co-parenting with an addicted mother can further complicate the trust-building process. It is crucial for moms in recovery to understand their legal rights and responsibilities. Seeking legal advice and working with a mediator can help navigate these complex situations, ensuring the best interests of the children are prioritized. By being proactive and transparent in legal proceedings, moms can demonstrate their dedication to their children's well-being.

Rebuilding trust with loved ones is a gradual process that requires patience, consistency, and open communication. By acknowledging the impact of addiction on family dynamics, seeking support for children, actively participating in recovery programs, and addressing legal and custody issues, moms in recovery can lay the foundation for healing and rebuilding trust with their loved ones. Through this journey, moms can not only regain the trust of their children but also strengthen their co-parenting relationships and create a healthier and more stable environment for their families.

Establishing Boundaries and Healthy Communication

One of the most crucial aspects of recovery for moms struggling with addiction is learning how to establish boundaries and maintain healthy communication. This subchapter aims to provide essential insights and practical strategies for moms in recovery who are navigating the challenges of co-parenting, dealing with custody issues, and supporting their children.

For moms in recovery, it is essential to recognize the significance of setting boundaries. This involves clearly defining and communicating personal limits to ensure a healthy and safe environment for both themselves and their children. By establishing boundaries, moms can protect their recovery journey and create a stable foundation for their families. This subchapter will delve into various techniques for setting boundaries effectively with co-parents, family members, and friends.

Furthermore, healthy communication is vital for maintaining harmonious relationships, especially when co-parenting with an addicted mother. Effective communication can help build trust, foster understanding, and ensure the well-being of the children involved. This subchapter will explore strategies for improving communication skills, such as active listening, assertive communication, and conflict resolution techniques. It will also provide guidance on how to address challenging conversations, discuss addiction-related concerns, and collaborate on important decisions.

In addition to addressing the needs of moms in recovery, this subchapter will also provide valuable insights for individuals in various niches. For instance, "My Daughter's Mom is a Junkie" offers guidance on how to support and protect children growing up with an addicted mother, emphasizing coping strategies, open dialogue, and emotional support. "Coping Strategies for Children with Addicted Parents" provides practical advice for children dealing with the challenges of addiction within their families, such as self-care, seeking support, and expressing emotions.

Furthermore, this subchapter will shed light on addiction recovery programs specifically tailored for mothers. It will outline available resources, treatment options, and support groups that cater to the specific needs of moms in recovery. Additionally, it will touch upon legal and custody issues in co-parenting scenarios with an addicted mother, offering guidance on navigating the legal system and ensuring the best interests of the children involved.

By focusing on establishing boundaries and healthy communication, this subchapter aims to empower moms in recovery, assist children coping with addiction in their families, provide insights into tailored recovery programs, and shed light on legal and custody matters. Ultimately, it seeks to support moms in their journey towards sustained recovery and the creation of a healthier and happier life for themselves and their families.

Chapter 7: Maintaining Long-Term Recovery as a Mom

Relapse Prevention Strategies

As a mom in recovery, one of the most important aspects of maintaining your sobriety is having effective relapse prevention strategies in place. Relapse can be a setback, but with the right tools and support, you can stay on track and continue your journey towards a healthier and happier life.

1. Building a Support Network: Surrounding yourself with a strong support system is crucial. Connect with other moms in recovery, join

support groups, or seek out a sponsor who can provide guidance and accountability. Having people who understand your struggles and can offer encouragement will greatly reduce the risk of relapse.

2. Self-Care: Taking care of yourself is essential for maintaining sobriety. Prioritize your physical, emotional, and mental well-being. Engage in activities that bring you joy and help you relax, such as exercise, meditation, or hobbies. By nurturing yourself, you are better equipped to handle stress and avoid triggers that may lead to relapse.

3. Identifying Triggers: It's important to recognize the people, places, and situations that may tempt you to use substances again. Identify your triggers and develop strategies to cope with them. This could involve avoiding certain environments, establishing healthy boundaries with toxic relationships, or finding alternative ways to manage stress and emotions.

4. Developing Coping Skills: Find healthy coping mechanisms to replace the urge to use drugs or alcohol. This could include practicing mindfulness, deep breathing exercises, journaling, or engaging in creative outlets. Explore different coping strategies until you find what works best for you.

5. Relapse Prevention Plan: Create a personalized relapse prevention plan that outlines your triggers, coping mechanisms, and steps to take in case of a potential relapse. This plan should incorporate emergency contacts, crisis hotlines, and professional resources that can provide immediate assistance during challenging times.

By implementing these relapse prevention strategies, you can navigate the challenges of recovery while being the best mom possible for your child. Remember, your journey is unique, and it's okay to ask for help when needed. Seeking addiction recovery programs specifically tailored for mothers can provide you with valuable resources and support.

Additionally, it's important to address legal and custody issues that may arise when co-parenting with an addicted mother. Consult with legal professionals or support groups that specialize in this area to ensure the best interests of your child are protected.

For moms whose children are coping with addicted parents, it's crucial to provide them with coping strategies. Open, honest communication is key. Help your child understand addiction in an age-appropriate way, and offer them a safe space to express their feelings and concerns. Encourage them to engage in activities they enjoy and surround them with positive role models who can offer guidance and support.

Remember, recovery is a journey, and relapse does not define your worth or strength as a mother. With determination, support, and the right strategies in place, you can overcome addiction and create a bright future for yourself and your child.

Self-Care for Mothers in Recovery

As a mom in recovery, it is crucial to prioritize self-care in order to maintain your own well-being and provide the best support for your children. This subchapter will explore various aspects of self-care and provide practical tips and strategies to help you navigate this important journey.

First and foremost, it is essential to acknowledge and celebrate your progress in recovery. Be proud of yourself for taking the courageous step towards a healthier and happier life. Remember that self-care is not selfish, it is an essential part of maintaining your sobriety and overall wellness.

One aspect of self-care is maintaining a healthy lifestyle. This includes eating nutritious meals, exercising regularly, and getting enough sleep. Physical activity can help reduce stress, boost your mood, and increase your overall energy levels. Additionally, ensuring that you are getting enough rest and fueling your body with nourishing foods will provide the energy you need to be present for your children.

Another important aspect of self-care is emotional well-being. Engaging in activities that bring you joy and relaxation is crucial for maintaining a balanced state of mind. Whether it's reading a book, practicing meditation or mindfulness, or pursuing a hobby, find activities that help you unwind and recharge.

Building a support network is also vital in your recovery journey. Seek out and connect with other mothers who have faced similar challenges. Online communities, support groups, and therapy sessions can provide a safe space to share experiences, gain insights, and receive much-needed encouragement.

Additionally, it is crucial to address any legal and custody issues that may arise in co-parenting with an addicted mother. Seek professional legal advice to ensure that you are aware of your rights and responsibilities, as well as the best course of action to protect your children's well-being.

Lastly, consider exploring addiction recovery programs specifically tailored for mothers. These programs often provide specialized support and address unique challenges that mothers in recovery may face. They can offer guidance on parenting, rebuilding relationships, and developing coping strategies.

Remember, self-care is an ongoing journey that requires dedication and commitment. By prioritizing your own well-being, you can become a stronger and more resilient mother, providing your children with the love and support they need. Embrace self-care as an essential part of your recovery and enjoy the rewards it brings to both you and your family.

In the next subchapter, we will address coping strategies for children with addicted parents, providing valuable insights and practical tools to help your children navigate the challenges they may face.

Finding Support and Community

Recovering from addiction can be a challenging and isolating journey, especially for mothers who are trying to rebuild their lives while also taking care of their children. In this subchapter, we will explore the importance of finding support and community for moms in recovery. Whether you are a mom who is battling addiction or someone who is supporting a mom in recovery, understanding the various aspects of finding support is crucial for successful recovery. For moms who are battling addiction, it is essential to find a community of like-minded individuals who can provide empathy, understanding, and guidance. Connecting with other moms in recovery can be a powerful way to share experiences, exchange coping strategies, and build a network of support. Online forums, support groups, and local recovery meetings specifically tailored for mothers can offer a safe space to discuss the unique challenges of balancing motherhood and recovery.

Additionally, it is important for moms in recovery to address the impact of their addiction on their children. Coping strategies for children with addicted parents can help both moms and their children navigate this difficult situation. This subchapter will delve into effective strategies such as open communication, age-appropriate education about addiction, and seeking professional help if needed. By understanding the needs of their children and providing them with the necessary support, moms in recovery can foster a healthier environment for their families.

Furthermore, this subchapter will explore addiction recovery programs specifically tailored for mothers. These programs often provide specialized services such as childcare, parenting classes, and therapy sessions that address the unique challenges faced by moms in recovery. By participating in these programs, moms can gain the tools and skills needed to rebuild their lives and create a stable and nurturing environment for their children.

Lastly, legal and custody issues in co-parenting with an addicted mother can be complex and emotionally challenging. This subchapter will offer guidance on navigating these legal matters, including seeking professional advice, understanding the rights and responsibilities of all parties involved, and exploring options such as supervised visitation or custody arrangements that prioritize the well-being of the children.

In conclusion, finding support and community is vital for moms in recovery. By connecting with others who understand their journey, exploring coping strategies for children, participating in tailored recovery programs, and navigating legal and custody issues, moms can build a strong support system that will enhance their chances of successful recovery and improve the well-being of their families. Remember, you are not alone, and with the right support, you can overcome addiction and create a better future for yourself and your children.

Chapter 8: Thriving as a Mom in Recovery

Setting Goals and Pursuing Dreams

As a mom in recovery, you have already taken the first step towards reclaiming your life and creating a brighter future for yourself and your children. Now, it's time to focus on setting goals and pursuing your dreams. In this subchapter, we will explore the importance of goal setting, provide strategies for achieving your dreams, and address the unique challenges faced by moms in recovery.

Setting goals is essential for personal growth and long-term success. By defining what you want to achieve, you can create a roadmap to guide your journey. Start by reflecting on your passions, interests, and values. What are the dreams you've always had but never pursued due to addiction? Write them down and visualize yourself achieving them. This exercise will help you clarify your goals and ignite the motivation needed to pursue them.

However, pursuing dreams while in recovery can be challenging, especially when you have children to care for. Coping strategies for children with addicted parents will be crucial in ensuring their well-being while you focus on your goals. Prioritize open communication, establish routines, and provide a stable and loving environment.

Seek support from therapists, support groups, or addiction recovery programs specifically tailored for mothers. These resources will equip you with coping skills and strategies to navigate the challenges of parenthood while maintaining your recovery.

Legal and custody issues may also arise when co-parenting with an addicted mother. It is essential to educate yourself about your rights and responsibilities. Consulting with a family lawyer who specializes in addiction-related cases can provide valuable guidance. Remember, prioritizing your recovery and maintaining a healthy environment for your children are crucial factors that will influence custody decisions.

As you embark on your journey, remember that recovery is a lifelong process. Be patient with yourself and celebrate even the smallest victories. Set realistic and attainable goals, breaking them down into manageable steps. Surround yourself with a supportive network of friends, family, and fellow moms in recovery. Share your dreams and aspirations with them, as they can provide encouragement, accountability, and valuable insights.

In conclusion, setting goals and pursuing dreams is an integral part of the recovery journey for moms. By defining your aspirations, prioritizing your children's well-being, and seeking the necessary support, you can build a future filled with love, joy, and fulfillment. Remember, you are not alone in this battle. Together, we can overcome addiction and create a better life for ourselves and our children.

Embracing a Healthy Lifestyle

In the journey of addiction recovery, it is crucial for moms to embrace a healthy lifestyle not only for their own well-being but also for the well-being of their children. This subchapter is dedicated to exploring the various aspects of living a healthy and balanced life while navigating the challenges of addiction recovery.

One of the key areas that moms in recovery should focus on is self-care. It is essential to prioritize your physical, mental, and emotional health. This includes adopting healthy eating habits, regular exercise routines, and practicing stress management techniques such as meditation or journaling. Taking care of yourself not only helps you stay strong during your recovery but also sets an example for your children to prioritize their well-being.

In addition to self-care, establishing healthy boundaries is crucial in maintaining a balanced lifestyle. It is important to communicate openly and honestly with your children about your addiction and recovery journey. By setting clear boundaries, you can ensure a safe and stable environment for your children and help them understand the importance of boundaries in their own lives.

Furthermore, this subchapter delves into coping strategies for children with addicted parents. It addresses the unique challenges that children face when their mother is battling addiction. From explaining addiction in an age-appropriate manner to providing emotional support, moms in recovery will find valuable insights and practical tips to help their children cope with the effects of addiction.

Moreover, this subchapter explores addiction recovery programs specifically tailored for mothers. It provides an overview of various programs, support groups, and resources available to help moms in their recovery journey. These specialized programs not only address the addiction itself but also provide support for the unique challenges faced by mothers, including parenting while in recovery.

Lastly, legal and custody issues in co-parenting with an addicted mother are discussed in this subchapter. It provides guidance on navigating the legal system, understanding custody arrangements, and ensuring the best interests of the children. This information aims to empower moms in recovery to advocate for themselves and their children while dealing with legal complexities.

Embracing a healthy lifestyle is a vital component of addiction recovery for moms. By focusing on self-care, establishing boundaries, supporting children, accessing tailored recovery programs, and addressing legal issues, moms in recovery can create a stable and nurturing environment for themselves and their children. This subchapter aims to equip moms with the knowledge and tools necessary to embrace a healthy lifestyle while overcoming the challenges of addiction.

Celebrating Milestones and Successes

In the journey of addiction recovery, it is crucial to take a moment and acknowledge the milestones and successes along the way. For moms in recovery, these accomplishments are not only personal victories but also demonstrate the strength and resilience that can inspire others facing similar challenges. This subchapter will explore the importance of celebrating milestones and successes, providing guidance and encouragement for moms navigating the path of recovery.

One of the most significant milestones in the recovery journey is the decision to seek help and embark on the path to sobriety. It takes immense courage and determination to confront addiction head-on, and moms in recovery should be proud of taking that crucial step. By acknowledging this milestone, they can affirm their commitment to a healthier and more fulfilling life for themselves and their children.

As moms progress through their recovery, it is essential to recognize and celebrate the small victories along the way. These might include completing a certain number of days without substance use, successfully attending therapy or support group sessions, or reaching personal goals related to education or employment. By acknowledging these achievements, moms can build motivation, self-confidence, and a sense of accomplishment, which are vital for long-term recovery.

Moreover, celebrating milestones and successes can have a profound impact on the well-being of children with addicted parents. By witnessing their mother's progress and taking part in the festivities, children can gain a sense of hope, stability, and optimism for the future. This subchapter will provide coping strategies for children with addicted parents, emphasizing the importance of open communication, providing age-appropriate explanations, and fostering a supportive environment where children can express their emotions.

Additionally, this subchapter will shed light on addiction recovery programs specifically tailored for mothers. It will explore various treatment options, such as residential programs with childcare facilities or outpatient programs that accommodate the responsibilities of motherhood. By providing information on these specialized programs, moms in recovery can find the support they need to navigate the challenges of parenting while focusing on their own recovery.

Lastly, this subchapter will address legal and custody issues in co-parenting with an addicted mother. It will offer guidance on navigating the legal system, accessing resources for custody arrangements, and maintaining a healthy co-parenting relationship. By addressing these concerns, moms in recovery can ensure the well-being of their children and establish a stable and supportive environment for their continued growth and success.

In conclusion, celebrating milestones and successes is a crucial aspect of the journey to addiction recovery for moms. By acknowledging and rejoicing in these achievements, moms can build motivation, self-confidence, and inspire hope in others. This subchapter will provide guidance on celebrating milestones, coping strategies for children, specialized recovery programs for mothers, and legal and custody issues in co-parenting. Through these insights, moms in recovery can find the support and encouragement they need to navigate the challenges they face and create a brighter future for themselves and their families.

Conclusion: Embracing the Journey of Recovery as a Mom

Congratulations! You have come to the end of this guide, "The Addiction Battle: A Guide for Moms in Recovery," and you should be proud of yourself for embarking on this challenging but rewarding journey of recovery. As a mom in recovery, you have shown immense strength and determination, not only for yourself but also for the well-being of your children.

Throughout this book, we have explored various aspects of addiction, recovery, and the unique challenges that come with being a mother in this situation. From understanding the impact of addiction on your children to coping strategies, recovery programs, and legal issues, you have gained valuable knowledge and tools to navigate through this difficult path.

One of the most important aspects of your recovery journey is to acknowledge that it is a lifelong process. Recovery is not a destination but a continuous journey of growth and self-discovery. As a mom in recovery, it is crucial to embrace this journey and understand that it will have ups and downs, but each step forward is a victory.

Your children are an integral part of this journey, and it is important to involve them in an age-appropriate manner. They may have witnessed or experienced the consequences of addiction, and providing them with a safe space to express their feelings and concerns is vital. By openly communicating with your children about your recovery, you can help them understand addiction and its impact while assuring them of your commitment to change. Additionally, seeking support from addiction recovery programs specifically tailored for mothers can be highly beneficial. These programs offer a nurturing and understanding environment where you can connect with other moms in similar situations. Sharing your experiences, challenges, and successes with others can provide a sense of belonging and encouragement.

Legal and custody issues may also arise as you navigate your recovery journey. It is important to educate yourself about your rights and options, seeking legal advice if necessary. Co-parenting with an addicted mother can be complex, but with the right support and guidance, it is possible to establish healthy boundaries and provide a stable environment for your children.

Remember, recovery is a process that requires self-compassion and patience. Be kind to yourself, celebrate your achievements, and seek help when needed. You are not alone in this journey, and there are countless resources available to support you.

As a mom in recovery, you have the power to break the cycle of addiction and provide a brighter future for both yourself and your children. Embrace the journey, stay committed to your recovery, and know that you are capable of creating a life filled with love, joy, and fulfillment. You are an inspiration, and your resilience will be a guiding light for your children as they witness your transformation.